20 Questions & Answers About Ulcerative Colitis

Francis A. Farraye, MD, MSc
Clinical Director, Section of Gastroenterology
Boston Medical Center
Professor of Medicine
Boston University School of Medicine
Boston, MA

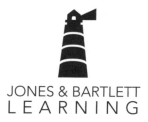

JONES & BARTLETT
LEARNING

World Headquarters
Jones & Bartlett Learning
40 Tall Pine Drive
Sudbury, MA 01776
978-443-5000
info@jblearning.com
www.jblearning.com

Jones & Bartlett Learning
Canada
6339 Ormindale Way
Mississauga, Ontario L5V 1J2
Canada

Jones & Bartlett Learning
International
Barb House, Barb Mews
London W6 7PA
United Kingdom

Jones & Bartlett Learning books and products are available through most bookstores and online booksellers. To contact Jones & Bartlett Learning directly, call 800-832-0034, fax 978-443-8000, or visit our website, www.jblearning.com.

The author, editor, and publisher have made every effort to provide accurate information. However, they are not responsible for errors, omissions, or for any outcomes related to the use of the contents of this book and take no responsibility for the use of the products and procedures described. Treatments and side effects described in this book may not be applicable to all people; likewise, some people may require a dose or experience a side effect that is not described herein. Drugs and medical devices are discussed that may have limited availability controlled by the Food and Drug Administration (FDA) for use only in a research study or clinical trial. Research, clinical practice, and government regulations often change the accepted standard in this field. When consideration is being given to use of any drug in the clinical setting, the healthcare provider or reader is responsible for determining FDA status of the drug, reading the package insert, and reviewing prescribing information for the most up-to-date recommendations on dose, precautions, and contraindications, and determining the appropriate usage for the product. This is especially important in the case of drugs that are new or seldom used.

Production Credits
Executive Publisher: Christopher Davis
Managing Editor for Custom Projects:
  Kathy Richardson
Associate Production Editor: Leah Corrigan
Marketing Manager: Rebecca Rockel
Manufacturing and Inventory Control
  Supervisor: Amy Bacus
Composition: Glyph International
Cover Design: Kate Ternullo

Cover Images (from left): © Monkey Business Images/ShutterStock, Inc., © Andy Lim/ShutterStock, Inc., © Kirk Peart Professional Imaging/ShutterStock, Inc., © NorthGeorgiaMedia/ShutterStock, Inc.
Photo Research and Permissions
  Manager: Kimberly Potvin
Printing and Binding: Malloy, Inc.
Cover Printing: Malloy, Inc.

ISBN-978-0-7637-9394-4

6048

Printed in the United States of America
14 13 12   10 9 8 7 6 5 4 3 2

This book is written for my patients with inflammatory bowel disease. It is dedicated to my loving and devoted family: my wife, Renee M. Remily, MD; my children, Jennifer and Alexis Farraye; and my parents, who taught me that hard work, perseverance, and commitment can result in great accomplishments.

Contents

PART ONE

The Basics

What are the inflammatory bowel diseases?

What is ulcerative colitis?

What are the symptoms of ulcerative colitis?

What is the difference between irritable bowel
syndrome and inflammatory bowel disease?

1. What are the inflammatory bowel diseases?

The **inflammatory bowel diseases (IBD)** include diseases of the large and **small intestines**, such as **ulcerative colitis (UC)** and **Crohn's disease (CD)**. While Crohn's disease can affect any part of the **gastrointestinal (GI)** tract, UC affects the **large intestine**, also called the **colon** (see **Figure 1**). In some people with UC involving the entire colon, the last 1 to 2 inches of the small intestine may also be involved. There are other types of **inflammation** in the colon, including infectious colitis, **ischemic colitis**, and **diverticulitis**. This book, however, focuses on questions about UC, which was first described in 1859, more than 150 years ago.

Inflammatory bowel disease (IBD)

Long-lasting disorders that cause inflammation in the gastrointestinal tract.

Small intestines

Organ where most digestion occurs. It measures about 20 feet and includes the duodenum, jejunum, and ileum.

Ulcerative colitis (UC)

Disease that causes ulcers and irritation in the inner lining of the colon and rectum.

Crohn's disease (CD)

Form of inflammatory bowel disease that causes inflammation in the gastrointestinal (GI) tract. It usually affects the lower small intestine or the colon, but it can also affect any part of the GI tract. Also called regional enteritis and ileitis.

Large intestine

Part of the intestine that includes the appendix, cecum, colon, and rectum. The large intestine absorbs water from the stool and changes it from a liquid to a solid form.

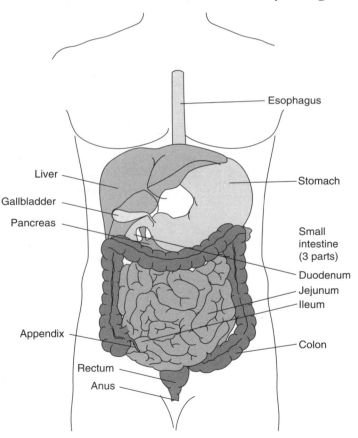

Figure 1   Normal gastrointestinal anatomy.

2. What is ulcerative colitis?

Ulcerative (meaning sores or **ulcers**) *colitis* (meaning inflammation of the colon) can involve any part of the large intestine. The inflammation always starts in the rectum and in some individuals it can extend upward into the colon. Although there are several layers that make up the colon, the inflammation in individuals with UC involves only the innermost lining called the **mucosa**. Ulcers or sores develop in the lining of the colon (see **Figures 2** and **3**). UC can involve the entire colon or just a small part of it. The different types of UC are based on how far they extend into the colon:

- **Ulcerative proctitis** is inflammation limited to the **rectum**.
- Ulcerative **proctosigmoiditis** involves the rectum and **sigmoid colon**.
- Inflammation that extends from the rectum, along the area above the sigmoid colon, up to the **splenic flexure** is called **left-sided colitis**.

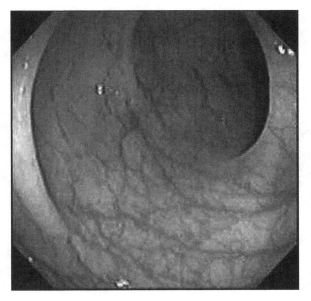

Figure 2   Normal colon as seen during colonoscopy.

Colon

Part of the large intestine extending from the cecum to, but not including, the rectum. *See Large intestine.*

Inflammation

Soreness, irritation, swelling.

Ischemic colitis

Irritation of the colon caused by decreased blood flow. It may cause bloody diarrhea.

Diverticulitis

Condition that occurs when small pouches in the colon called diverticula become inflamed.

Ulcer

Sore on the skin's surface or on the stomach or intestinal lining.

Mucosa

Lining of gastrointestinal tract organs that absorb nutrients and fluid, form a barrier, and produce mucus.

Ulcerative proctitis

Ulcerative colitis that occurs in the rectum.

Rectum

Lower end of the large intestine leading to the anus.

Proctosigmoiditis

Inflammation of the rectum and sigmoid colon.

The Basics

3

Sigmoid colon

Lower part of the colon that empties into the rectum.

Splenic flexure

Sharp bend between the transverse and descending colon in the left-upper quadrant of the abdomen.

Left-sided colitis

Inflammation that extends from the rectum to the area above the sigmoid colon to the splenic flexure.

Pancolitis

Inflammation that extends from the rectum and proximal to the splenic flexure.

Ileum

Lower end of the small intestine.

- Inflammation that extends above the splenic flexure is called **pancolitis** (sometimes called total colitis).
- Inflammation can spread into the last one to two inches of the small intestine (**ileum**) in individuals with pancolitis and this is called **backwash ileitis**.

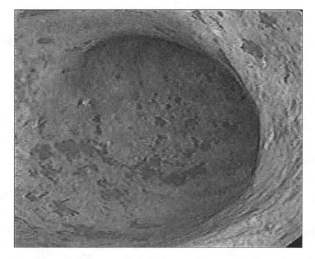

Figure 3   Colon with characteristic inflammation seen in ulcerative colitis.

Figure 4 shows some of these different types of UC. Studies in large populations of patients with UC show that about 30% have limited proctitis, about 30% have

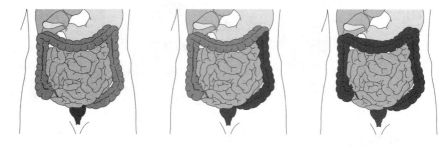

| Proctitis | Left-Sided Colitis | Pancolitis |

Figure 4   The three most common patterns of ulcerative colitis.

extensive UC or pancolitis, and about 40% have left-sided colitis. Over time, some patients who are initially diagnosed with a limited form of the disease like **proctitis** may begin to develop inflammation in other areas of the colon, leading to one of the more extensive forms of the disease.

There is no medical cure for UC, but most people can get effective treatment for their symptoms. There are medications that can be used to treat and manage UC (see Part 4), and some patients may need surgery (see Part 6). Ulcerative colitis is a lifelong condition and there are ways to cope with it beyond just taking pills (see Part 8).

It has been estimated that patients with UC account for 250,000 physician visits, 30,000 hospitalizations, and loss of over a million workdays per year. Furthermore, the direct medical costs of UC exceed $4 billion dollars annually. This includes over $960 million for hospital costs and $680 million for drug costs.

3. What are the symptoms of ulcerative colitis?

The most common symptom of UC is bloody **diarrhea**. Typically, a patient will first experience **abdominal** (stomach) discomfort, which will be followed by the bloody diarrhea (also referred to as "passing loose **stools**," which contain blood and **mucus**). The patient may feel an "**urgency**" about their need to find a toilet quickly. As the colitis gets worse, a patient may develop fatigue, fever, chills, loss of appetite, and weight loss. These symptoms help healthcare providers define colitis as "mild," "moderate," or "severe." The healthcare provider looks at a number of factors, including frequency of

Backwash ileitis
Inflammation of the last few inches of the small intestine in patients with pancolitis.

Proctitis
Inflammation of the rectum or anus.

Ulcerative colitis is a lifelong condition and there are ways to cope with it beyond just taking pills.

Diarrhea
Frequent, loose, and watery bowel movements. Causes include gastrointestinal infections, irritable bowel syndrome, inflammatory bowel disease, medicines, and malabsorption.

Abdominal
Related to the area between the chest and the hips containing the stomach, small intestine, large intestine, liver, gallbladder, pancreas, and spleen.

The Basics

5

Stool

Solid waste that passes through the rectum as a bowel movement; includes undigested food, bacteria, mucus, and dead cells. Also called *feces*.

Mucus

Clear liquid made by the intestines that coats and protects tissues in the gastrointestinal tract.

Urgency

Feeling of "needing to go" (either urine or stool).

Toxicity

The degree to which a substance can be harmful.

ESR

Erythrocyte sedimentation rate, a blood test that indicates inflammation in the body; it does not specify the location of the inflammation.

Anemia

Decreased red blood cells.

Fulminant

Rapidly developing and severe condition.

Distension

Stretched, expanded, or swollen out of shape.

diarrhea and signs of **toxicity** (fever, rapid heart rate, and abnormal lab tests). The categories of ulcerative colitis are usually determined as:

* *Mild*: When a patient has fewer than 4 stools daily (with or without blood), no related signs of toxicity, and a normal **erythrocyte sedimentation rate (ESR-** a blood test that indicates inflammation in the body).
* *Moderate*: When a patient has more than 4 stools daily but has minimal signs of toxicity.
* *Severe*: When a patient has 6 or more bloody stools per day and shows evidence of toxicity with a fever, rapid heart rate, **anemia,** and a higher-than-normal erythrocyte sedimentation rate (ESR).
* *Fulminant*: The most severe form of this disease is when the patient has more than 10 stools a day, experiences continuous rectal bleeding, abdominal pain and **distension**, blood transfusion requirement, and x-rays of the abdomen show distention of the colon.

The severity of the patient's symptoms is related to the extent of the inflammation in the colon (that is, the more severe the inflammation is, the worse the symptoms are). Patients can also have symptoms that involve their joints, skin, eyes, and liver. Symptoms of UC can come and go. When the UC symptoms are active, the patient is said to be having a "**flare**." When the symptoms seem to go away for a while, the patient is in "**remission**." Approximately 65–75% of patients with UC have what is called **chronic** intermittent UC characterized by periods of remission and disease activity. About 5–15% of individuals will have constant UC with symptoms present at all times. Another 10–25% of individuals will have only a single episode. In this latter group, it's possible that an undiagnosed infection presented with symptoms similar to UC.

4. What is the difference between irritable bowel syndrome and inflammatory bowel disease?

Although the names **irritable bowel syndrome (IBS)** and IBD sound alike, they are very different conditions. Irritable bowel syndrome is much more common than IBD. In fact, an estimated 15% of the U.S. population has symptoms of IBS.

Patients with IBS have some similar symptoms as those with UC. These include diarrhea, crampy abdominal pain, and **bloating**. However, unlike UC, patients with IBS do not usually have weight loss, **rectal bleeding** (unless they also have bleeding hemorrhoids), fever, anemia, or symptoms that wake them at night. In addition, patients with IBS do not have the **extra-intestinal** (outside the intestines) symptoms that can sometimes happen with UC, such as eye problems or mouth and skin ulcers. On the other hand, patients with IBS can develop a painful non-inflammatory joint and tissue condition called **fibromyalgia**.

Overall, diagnosing and managing patients with UC can be difficult if they also have IBS. UC affects men and women equally; IBS is nearly three times as common in women as it is in men. In particular it may be more difficult to differentiate between CD and IBS based on symptoms alone. **Table 1** lists some of the similarities and differences between UC and IBS.

Flare
Worsening of symptoms of disease.

Remission
Period of time when disease does not cause symptoms.

Chronic
Lasting for a long time

Irritable bowel syndrome (IBS)
Disorder associated with abdominal pain, bloating, and altered bowel habits. Also sometimes called *spastic colon* or *mucous colitis*.

Bloating
A fullness or swelling in the abdomen.

Rectal bleeding
Bleeding that originates in the rectum and comes out through the anus.

Extra-intestinal
Occurring outside of the intestines.

Fibromyalgia
Chronic illness characterized by fatigue and widespread aching of muscles and soft tissues.

The Basics

Table 1   Similarities and Differences between UC and IBS

	UC	IBS
Symptoms in common	Diarrhea, crampy abdominal pain, and bloating	Diarrhea, crampy abdominal pain, and bloating
Different symptoms	Weight loss, rectal bleeding, fever, anemia, nocturnal symptoms; symptoms and findings related to the eyes, liver, skin, and joints	Not typically seen in IBS patients
Gender	Affects men and women equally	70% women, 30% men
Colonoscopy findings	Inflammation and/or ulcers	No visible inflammation
Pathology	Biopsies show inflammation with crypt abscesses, crypt branching	No inflammation seen
Treatments	AZA/6-MP, balsalazide, mesalamine, sulfasalazine, biologics, ciprofloxacin, cyclosporine, metronidazole, methotrexate, steroids, surgery	Diet, antispasmodics, tricyclics, lubiprostone, alosetron; no surgery
Pattern of illness	Periods of active disease (flare) and periods of remission	Symptoms can come and go

PART TWO

Risk, Prevention, and Epidemiology

Who gets ulcerative colitis? How many people have ulcerative colitis in the United States?

Does ulcerative colitis run in families? Can I pass ulcerative colitis to my children?

What factors can affect ulcerative colitis?

5. Who gets ulcerative colitis? How many people have ulcerative colitis in the United States?

Both men and women can develop UC, and there are approximately 700,000 individuals in the United States living with the disease. The average age of onset of UC is between the ages of 15 and 25 years, but it can be diagnosed at any age. Approximately 30,000 new cases of UC and Crohn's disease are diagnosed yearly. For every 100,000 individuals, 10 to 12 new cases of UC are diagnosed each year, and studies show that this number has been rising over the past 10 years.

Although anyone can get UC, there are certain groups of people who are more likely to develop this disease. White individuals develop UC more commonly than other racial groups. Individuals of Jewish descent, especially of northern European origin, are 3 to 5 times more likely to be affected by IBD. IBD is more common in the United States and Europe and less common in the developing countries of Africa and South America. However, even geographic areas where the incidence of IBD is low have seen increases in the number of new cases.

6. Does ulcerative colitis run in families? Can I pass ulcerative colitis to my children?

Yes, UC does run in families. As many as 1 in 5 individuals with UC have a family member who also has UC. Research shows that 10% of identical twins will develop UC. Despite having the same **genetic** profile, the fact that only 1 in 10 sets of identical twins both develop UC stresses the point that environmental exposures play an important role in the development of UC. Currently, there is no way to predict if a particular

Genetic

Relating to biologic inheritance.

family member will develop UC; however, if you have UC, there is an increased chance that your children, brothers, and sisters will also develop the disease. Although there is no testing presently available for a specific UC gene that predicts if your children will get UC, the risk to your children has been estimated to be 8%, though higher rates have been reported in certain ethnic groups. Despite this increased risk, you should not dismiss the idea of having children.

7. What factors can affect ulcerative colitis?

There are several things that can affect flare-ups in UC. For instance, there is a class of drugs called nonsteroidal anti-inflammatory drugs (**NSAIDs**), which are used by many people to treat aches and pain (including headaches, and menstrual-related pain). Common NSAIDs include aspirin, naproxen, and ibuprofen. Some patients with UC can experience a flare of their colitis when taking NSAIDs. However, low-dose aspirin (81 mg) is felt to be safe. This class of drugs can sometimes cause upper abdominal discomfort and internal bleeding, in addition to other side effects. On the other hand, acetaminophen can be taken safely by patients with UC. If you do need to take a NSAID, consider taking the lowest possible dose, take it with food, and take it for the shortest period of time possible. Please talk to your doctor to determine what is best for you. Some studies suggest that use of the acne drug isotretinoin may be associated with the development of IBD. Please talk with your healthcare provider to determine what is best for you.

Interestingly, people who smoke are less likely to have UC, and it has been well established that individuals can develop UC after they stop smoking. However, the multiple negative effects of smoking far outweigh any

Risk, Prevention, and Epidemiology

NSAID
Nonsteroidal anti-inflammatory drug, such as aspirin, ibuprofen, and naproxen.

Lactose intolerance

Being unable to digest lactose, the sugar in milk. This condition occurs when the body cannot produce lactase.

Celiac disease

Immune reaction to gluten, a protein found in wheat, rye, and barley. The disease causes damage to the lining of the small intestine and prevents absorption of nutrients. Also called *celiac sprue*, *gluten intolerance*, and *nontropical sprue*.

Gluten

Protein found in wheat, rye, and barley. In people with celiac disease, gluten damages the lining of the small intestine or causes sores on the skin. See *Celiac disease*.

Colorectal cancer

Cancer that starts in the colon (also called the *large intestine*) or the rectum (the end of the large intestine).

benefit in managing UC. A healthcare provider may consider treating an ex-smoker with a nicotine patch, which appears to have some benefit.

Although many patients feel that their diet plays a role in their colitis, there is no evidence to support that a specific diet can cause intestinal inflammation. Certainly when your colitis is active, following a low-fiber diet is suggested.

All individuals, regardless of UC, are encouraged to eat a well-balanced diet. If certain foods seem to increase diarrhea or abdominal pain, consider eliminating each food individually on a trial basis. Some individuals can have **lactose intolerance** in addition to UC. Finally, patients with UC have an increased risk of **celiac disease** (allergy to **gluten**), and should be tested for this disorder if symptoms are ongoing. A consultation with a nutritionist can be helpful.

As with diet, stress can cause many gastrointestinal symptoms but there is no evidence to support that stress causes UC. If a patient who feels stress in their life and is unable to cope with a UC diagnosis, their healthcare provider may have some helpful insight. See Question 17 about healthy coping and stress management.

Talk to your healthcare provider about the importance of staying on medications, even when you are feeling well. Continued medication use may increase the chance of remaining in remission and may lower the risk of developing **colorectal cancer**.

PART THREE

Diagnosis

How is the diagnosis of ulcerative colitis made?

Do I have Crohn's Disease? How can I tell if it is Crohn's Disease?

8. How is the diagnosis of ulcerative colitis made?

Because loose, bloody stools can have other causes, your clinician will typically obtain stool samples to make sure there is no evidence of an infection that can mimic UC. Common bacteria that can cause infections leading to bloody diarrhea include *Salmonella, Shigella, Campylobacter*, and *E. coli* 0157. Rarely are bloody stools caused by a parasite or infection with *C. difficile*, a bacteria commonly associated with taking antibiotics and often acquired in hospitals. You don't need to travel to exotic places in the world to develop these infections: you can be exposed to them in nursing homes or restaurants. Stool samples are sent to a lab to determine if a bacterium is causing the diarrhea and examined to look for parasites and ova (eggs of the parasites).

A healthcare provider may refer a patient to a **gastroenterologist** if your diarrhea continues and the stool samples fail to identify an infection. The gastroenterologist will take a detailed history and perform a physical examination. He or she may ask about eye, skin, and joint symptoms, as these "extra-intestinal" symptoms can be present in patients with UC. In some situations, joint pain, skin lesions, and eye symptoms may occur even before abdominal pain and diarrhea begin.

Blood tests will be done to look for inflammation, certain types of proteins associated with IBD, and anemia caused by blood loss. These tests include the following:

- **CBC** (complete blood count)
- Comprehensive **metabolic panel** which evaluates liver and kidney functions
- ESR (erythrocyte sedimentation rate)
- **CRP** (C-reactive protein)

Gastroenterologist

Doctor who specializes in the diagnosis and treatment of digestive diseases.

CBC

Abbreviation for the blood test, complete blood count, which measures red cells and white cells.

Metabolic panel

Blood tests that measure sodium, potassium, chloride, bicarbonate, blood urea nitrogen (BUN), creatinine, and glucose.

CRP

C-reactive protein is a blood test that measures a type of protein found in blood associated with inflammatory diseases and risk of heart disease.

A complete blood count will be obtained to determine the white blood cell and red blood cell count. The white blood cell count can be higher in patients with colitis. Similarly, chronic intestinal bleeding can cause a lower red blood cell count and the patient can develop anemia. A comprehensive metabolic panel evaluates your liver and kidney function to make sure these organs are working correctly. Blood tests for erythrocyte sedimentation rate (ESR) and C-reactive protein (CRP) are usually done to look for signs of inflammation. In some situations, blood might be tested to measure for specific antibodies that are associated with UC.

Your gastroenterologist will then most likely perform a **sigmoidoscopy** or **colonoscopy** to examine the lining of your colon. A sigmoidoscopy is usually performed without **sedation** and uses a thin (about the size of your index finger) flexible tube with a light that is inserted into the rectum to examine the lower third of the colon. Preparation for a sigmoidoscopy requires the use of rectally-administered **enemas** that empty the **lower bowel**.

Patients are unable to have any solid food the day before your colonoscopy. A laxative is given the night before the procedure to cleanse the bowel of stool, which allows your physician to get good views of the colon. More recently, clinicians have begun using a "split" dose of bowel laxatives in which one dose is given the night before the procedure and one given early on the morning of your test. While the patient is lying on their left side, the gastroenterologist performs a rectal exam with a gloved and lubricated finger. The **colonoscope** (a long, flexible tube with a light and camera) is inserted into the anus and to the cecum and terminal ileum (see **Figure 5**). Although flexible sigmoidoscopy is typically performed without sedation,

Sigmoidoscopy

Looking into the sigmoid colon and rectum with a flexible or rigid tube called a sigmoidoscope.

Colonoscopy

Test to look into the rectum and colon that uses a long, flexible, narrow tube with a light and tiny camera on the end. The tube is called a **colonoscope**.

Sedation

Administration of medications during a test to reduce anxiety and discomfort.

Enemas

Insertion of a liquid into the rectum and lower colon as a treatment.

Lower bowel

Lower part of the colon that connects to the anus.

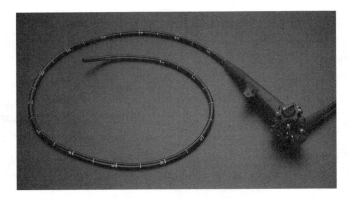

Figure 5   Colonoscope is the tube with a light and camera, which is inserted into the anus to see inside the colon.

Used with permission of Fujinon, Inc.

sedation is given in nearly all patients undergoing colonoscopy. Mild cramping may be felt during the procedure. Cramping can be reduced by taking several slow, deep breaths during the procedure. The gastroenterologist will also look for inflammation and abnormalities of the colon, such as **polyps** or ulcers. Tissue samples, called biopsies are obtained during the procedure. See **Figures 6** and **7**, which show a normal colon **biopsy** and one from a patient with UC.

Polyp

An abnormal growth on the surface of the intestine.

Biopsy

Procedure in which a tiny piece of a body part, such as the colon or liver, is removed for examination with a microscope.

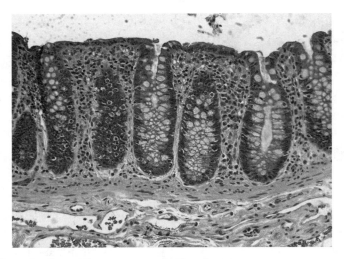

Figure 6   Normal tissue as seen under the microscope.

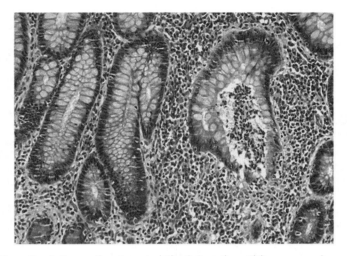

Figure 7   Inflammation characteristic of ulcerative colitis as seen under the microscope.

The biopsied material is sent to a pathologist who examines the tissue under a microscope. There are specific findings on the biopsy that can establish a diagnosis of IBD. Depending on the symptoms, the clinician might also order x-rays of the small intestine, such as an **upper GI series** with a **small bowel x-ray** or a **CT scan** of the abdomen. It is important that a diagnosis of UC be firmly established. Following the clinician's recommendation to have this testing will assist in proper diagnosis.

9. Do I have Crohn's Disease? How can I tell if it is Crohn's Disease?

Crohn's disease (CD) is the other major form of IBD. It affects approximately 700,000 Americans. Unlike UC, which affects the colon, Crohn's disease can affect the entire gastrointestinal tract (see **Figure 8**). CD is limited to the small intestine in 33% of patients and to the colon in 20% of patients. Both the large and the small intestines are affected in the majority of patients

Upper GI series

X-rays of the esophagus, stomach, and duodenum. The patient swallows barium before x-rays are taken. Barium makes the organs show up on x-rays.

Small bowel x-ray

X-rays of the small intestine taken as barium liquid passes through the organ. Also called *Small bowel follow-through.*

CT scan

Abbreviation for computed tomography, a technique of imaging body organs with detailed, cross-sectional views; can be done with or without oral and intravenous contrast dye.

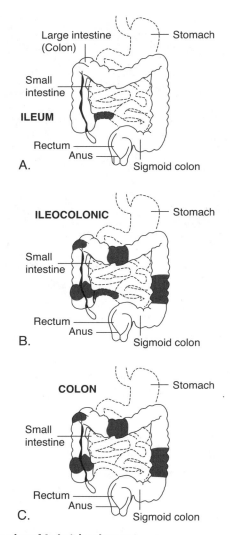

Figure 8   Location of Crohn's involvement.

Ileocolitis

Irritation of the lower part of the small intestine (ileum) and the beginning part of the colon.

Ileitis

Inflammation of the small intestine. Many different disorders can cause inflammation of the small intestine.

with Crohn's. CD most typically involves the small intestine and colon at the same time and is called **ileo-colitis**. Isolated inflammation of the small intestine is called **ileitis**. Isolated inflammation of the colon is called Crohn's colitis. Inflammation in Crohn's disease can be patchy with areas of normal tissue surrounded by areas of inflammation (skip areas).

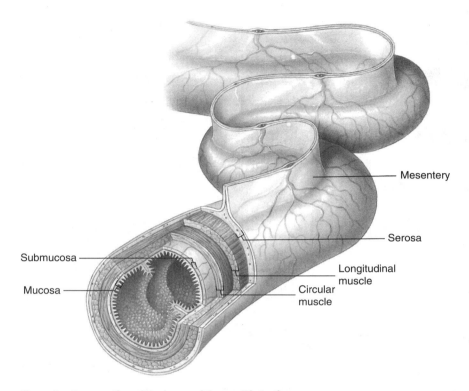

Mesentery

Serosa

Submucosa

Mucosa

Longitudinal muscle

Circular muscle

Figure 9   Cross-section of the layers of the small intestines.

There are several layers that make up the colon, and inflammation of UC and Crohn's disease involve different parts. The inflammation of UC involves only the innermost lining, called the **mucosa** (see Figure 9). However, CD can affect all layers of the colon. Because the ulcers from Crohn's can penetrate the entire wall of the intestine, a **fistula** and/or **abscess** can develop. Fistulas, which are abnormal connections between two organs, can develop next to the anus or between the intestine and adjacent organs, such as the bladder, vagina, or skin. Abscesses are collections of pus and can occur within the abdomen or around the anal area.

Fistula

Abnormal passage between two organs, or between an organ and the outside of the body, caused when inflamed tissues come into contact and join together while healing.

Abscess

Accumulation of pus.

19

MRI scan

A magnetic resonance imaging (MRI) scan is a test that uses a magnetic field and pulses of radio wave energy to make pictures of organs and structures inside the body.

Granulomatous colitis

Another name for Crohn's disease of the colon.

Granulomas

Finding seen under the microscope in some patients with Crohn's disease.

Indeterminate colitis

Inflammation of the colon that cannot be easily classified as either UC or CD.

There are also features found on colonoscopy and biopsy that can help gastroenterologists distinguish UC from CD. While UC always involves the rectum, the rectum is affected in only 10–20% of individuals with CD. X-rays of the abdomen can also help distinguish UC from CD. Such x-rays include an upper GI series with a small bowel x-ray and a CT scan of the abdomen and pelvis. **MRI scans** are being performed more frequently as an alternative to CT scans as there is no radiation exposure during a MRI. Although CD can involve the stomach and small intestines, UC does not. Another name for CD is **granulomatous colitis**. This is because under the microscope, **granulomas** are found in about 25% of patients with CD but not in patients with UC. Rectal bleeding is less common in patients with CD.

Table 2 shows a list of features that can be helpful in distinguishing UC from CD. Carefully listening to and analyzing symptoms, performing a physical exam, and using a combination of tests, typically enables the clinician to distinguish UC from CD. In about 10% of cases, it may be difficult to distinguish UC from CD of the colon; this is called **indeterminate colitis**.

There are also differences in the tissue biopsied from the affected part of the GI tract. See **Table 3** for an explanation of these differences.

Figure 7 shows what the biopsied tissue (in UC) looks like under the microscope.

Table 2   Clinical Differences between UC and Crohn's Disease

Clinical Characteristic	Ulcerative Colitis	Crohn's Disease
Diarrhea	Typical	Typical
Rectal bleeding	Typical	Occurs
Abdominal mass	Not seen	Occurs
Mucosal disease	Continuous from rectum	Patchy (skip lesions)
Pseudopolyps	Seen	Seen
Rectal involvement	Characteristic	Occurs
Fistula	Not seen	Occurs
Perianal disease	Not seen	Occurs
Toxic megacolon	Occurs	Rare
Small bowel involvement	Not seen	Common
Cancer	Occurs (colon)	Occurs
pANCA	60–70%	15%
pASCA	15%	65%

Table 3   Pathologic Differences between UC and Crohn's Disease

Pathologic Characteristic	Ulcerative Colitis	Crohn's Disease
Depth	Mucosal	Transmural (full thickness of the colon or small intestine)
Crypt abscesses	Seen	Seen
Architecture distortion	Seen	Seen
Granuloma	Not seen	Occurs
Linear ulcerations	Not seen	Occurs
Mesenteric fat, nodes	Not involved	Involved

PART FOUR

Treatment Options

What are the different types of medications
used to treat ulcerative colitis?

I am currently feeling well, so why do I have
to keep taking my medications?

5-ASAs

Aminosalicylates are medications used to treat the inflammation associated with ulcerative colitis; they come in oral and topical forms.

Immunomodulators

Class of drugs that are capable of modifying (decrease or weaken) the effectiveness of the immune system.

Corticosteroids

Class of medications given to reduce inflammation.

Biologic agents

Group of therapeutic medications that include monoclonal antibodies.

Immune system

Complex and intertwined system of cells and genetics that controls the body's defense system against infection and other foreign organisms or substances.

10. What are the different types of medications used to treat ulcerative colitis?

Several types ("classes") of medications are used to treat patients with UC. The major classes include the **5-ASAs, immunomodulators, corticosteroids,** and **biologic agents**.

The 5-ASA (Aminosalicylates) agents are usually taken by mouth and act to reduce inflammation, but do not affect the **immune system**. In addition to oral preparations, other 5-ASA treatments include **retention enemas** and **suppositories**.

Immunomodulators are used in patients who do not respond to anti-inflammatory medications (5-ASAs). Although these medications reduce the inflammation of UC, they (among other things) can also decrease the body's immune system functioning and increase the risk of infections. Patients on immunomodulators need regular monitoring of their blood to look for decreased red and white blood cells as well as elevation in the liver function tests (which are possible effects of the medications).

Like immunomodulators, corticosteroids also act on the immune system and are used in oral, rectal, and IV forms. Corticosteroids reduce the inflammation associated with UC and are in a class of drugs called anti-inflammatories. Although very effective for short-term use, there is a long list of side effects in patients chronically treated with corticosteroids.

Biologic agents are drugs that target specific proteins in the body. Some biologic agents block the production of **tumor necrosis factor (TNF)**. TNF is a protein that circulates in the blood and is associated with inflammation in the intestines.

Antibiotics are not routinely used to treat patients with UC; however, they are used to treat infections that may result from being on immunomodulators or corticosteroids.

Many individuals are using **prebiotics** and **probiotics** to treat IBD. Prebiotics are nondigestible nutrients that help promote the growth of "good" bacteria in your body. Probiotics are the actual "good" bacteria themselves in the form of a dietary supplement. Data supporting the use of prebiotics and probiotics is limited and they may not be covered by insurance.

In some situations, agents that help reduce the spasms of pain and the bouts of diarrhea are used in combination with the medications above to treat the symptoms of abdominal cramps and frequent loose stools.

Acetaminophen is the preferred pain medication for use in patients with UC. The chronic use of narcotic medications should be avoided, given the potential for addiction. Patients with chronic pain unrelated to active colitis might benefit from a referral to a comprehensive pain center.

11. I am currently feeling well, so why do I have to keep taking my medications?

Many patients with chronic disorders stop taking their medications for a period of time or miss doses, and studies show that 43–72% of patients with IBD do not take their medications as prescribed. There are many reasons why a person might stop taking their medication. Statistics show that those who stop are more likely to be male, single, have limited colitis, be taking rectally administered medications, or be prescribed multiple medications. Several research studies have demonstrated

Retention enema
Insertion of medicated fluids through the anus into the rectum and lower colon to allow the fluid to come in contact with the mucosal lining of the colon to help heal inflammation.

Suppositories
Small plug of medication inserted in the rectum.

Tumor necrosis factor (TNF)
Type of protein that promotes inflammation in the body and gastrointestinal tract.

Prebiotics
Nondigestible food ingredients that are ingested by the normal bacteria occurring in the colon. They are believed to aid in digestion.

Probiotics
Live beneficial bacteria found in food or diet supplements believed to aid in digestion.

Treatment Options

that patients with UC who do not take their medications are five times more likely to develop a flare of their colitis.

Aside from the discomfort of a flare-up, evidence suggests that severe colon inflammation seen on colonoscopy and/or on colon biopsies may increase risk of colitis relapse, need for surgery to remove the colon, or development of cancer. Because several of the commonly used UC medications work to heal the inner lining of the colon, it is not surprising that many healthcare providers feel that patients should stay on their medications even when they are well. Please talk with your healthcare provider before discontinuing any medication, to discuss the risks and benefits. There may be ways to change the medication routine to make it more convenient.

PART FIVE

Complications

What is my risk of developing colon cancer? Is there anything I can do to decrease my risk? How is chromoendoscopy used to diagnose colon cancer?

What is toxic megacolon?

12. What is my risk of developing colon cancer? Is there anything I can do to decrease my risk? How is chromoendoscopy used to diagnose colon cancer?

Colorectal cancer (CRC), which includes cancer of the colon and rectum, is one of the most feared complications of ulcerative colitis for patients and physicians alike. More than 135,000 cases of CRC are diagnosed annually in the United States, making it the second most common cancer. Patients with UC or Crohn's disease comprise 1–2% of new CRC cases.

It is important to note that the overwhelming majority of patients with UC will *not* develop colon cancer. In fact, recent studies suggest that the risk of developing colon cancer is significantly lower than previously thought. Patients who have had extensive UC for 20 years, you have a 2.5% risk of developing colon cancer; for 30 years have a 7.6% risk; and for 40 years have a 11% risk.

Patients with certain types of UC are however, at increased risk of developing colon cancer. The highest risk group includes patients with extensive UC or pancolitis. Patients with left-sided colitis are at an intermediate risk, but those with ulcerative proctitis or proctosigmoiditis are not at any higher risk than the general population.

The risk of developing CRC increases after approximately 8 years of disease. This timeline is based on the onset of symptoms, as opposed to the time when the diagnosis was made by a healthcare provider. The following are additional factors for a patient and their clinician to consider when assessing risk for CRC:

- Extent of colonic inflammation
- Severity of colonic inflammation
- Duration of UC from onset of symptoms
- Family history of colon cancer in parents, brothers, or sisters (**first-degree relatives**)
- A first-degree relative diagnosed with CRC younger than 50
- **Primary sclerosing cholangitis or PSC** (significantly increases risk of CRC)

At this time it is not clear if children diagnosed with UC are at an increased risk of developing CRC, compared to adults, given that children have UC for a longer time solely based on their age at diagnosis. It is suggested that children, like adults, should follow screening recommendations.

All patients should undergo a colonoscopy 8–10 years after the onset of symptoms of colitis. Biopsies will be taken throughout the colon. At that time, the extent of the disease can be determined based on the results of the biopsies and visual appearance of the lining of the colon. Typically, patients with more extensive colitis undergo colonoscopy every 1–3 years after their initial screening colonoscopy and 8–10 years after the onset of symptoms. The interval between colonoscopies depends on the number of risk factors described above; however, patients with primary sclerosing cholangitis should have a yearly colonoscopy once the diagnosis is made.

The good news is that the risk of developing CRC in patients with UC is decreasing. The lower risk may be related to widespread use of effective medical therapy, more frequent colonoscopies, and the use of **colectomy** in selected patients. Some individuals at higher risk for CRC may benefit from being in a surveillance program that includes regular colonoscopies.

First-degree relatives

Mother, father, sister, brother, son, or daughter.

Primary sclerosing cholangitis (PSC)

Irritation, scarring, and narrowing of the bile ducts inside and outside the liver. Bile builds up in the liver and may damage its cells. Many people with this condition also have ulcerative colitis.

Colectomy

A surgical procedure to remove all or part of the colon.

Complications

29

To decrease the risk of developing CRC, here are some things that UC patients can do:

- Be aware of risk factors
- Consult with a healthcare provider about remaining on medications to prevent **relapses** and control inflammation in the colon
- Comply with the schedule of colonoscopies as developed by a clinician

Chromoendoscopy

Procedure by which dye is sprayed on the lining of the colon to make it easier to identify abnormalities during a colonoscopy.

Chromoendoscopy is a technique used to detect abnormalities in the colon of patients with UC. As discussed previously, patients with extensive and long-standing UC have an increased risk of developing colorectal cancer (CRC). Presently, multiple random biopsies of the colon are obtained during colonoscopy to screen for CRC. Any suspicious abnormalities observed by the gastroenterologist are also biopsied during the colonoscopy.

Chromoendoscopy entails spraying the colon with a dye that stains the lining and allows a clinician to more easily identify suspicious areas and biopsy them. The staining is not permanent and has no lasting effect on the patient's colon. The two stains most commonly used are indigo carmine and methylene blue. Several studies have demonstrated that the colonoscopy and chromoendoscopy together can identify more serious abnormalities than random biopsies. Colonoscopy with chromoendoscopy may take more time than standard colonoscopy. At present, chromoendoscopy is reserved for patients at an increased risk of developing cancer or for those patients in whom suspicious findings were identified on earlier procedures.

Toxic megacolon

Life-threatening complication usually from IBD that results in dilatation of the colon and possible perforation; may require emergency surgery to remove the colon.

13. What is toxic megacolon?

Toxic megacolon is a serious and potentially life-threatening complication that can occur in patients with severe or fulminant UC. It can happen at any time after the diagnosis of UC, but it most frequently develops within several years of the initial UC diagnosis. Individuals who develop toxic megacolon are quite ill with fever, abdominal pain, and bloody stools. The white blood cell count is elevated and the patient is anemic. The heart rate becomes rapid and the blood pressure drops. X-rays show dilation of the colon.

Patients with toxic megacolon need careful observation by a gastroenterologist and surgeon. The patient is not allowed to eat anything, including liquids, and often a **nasogastric tube** is placed through the nose into the stomach to decompress the intestines. Medical therapy is given with intravenous fluids, corticosteroids and antibiotics. Bacterial infections should be excluded by stool testing. If the patient with toxic megacolon does not improve within 24–48 hours, emergency surgery is needed to remove the colon before it perforates (breaks open). While toxic megacolon may not be a frequent complication of severe UC, the risk of emergency surgery or even death makes it a serious complication. Patients who experience severe abdominal pain, especially if it accompanied by fever, bloody diarrhea, rapid heart rate, or abdominal tenderness, should contact their healthcare provider immediately.

Nasogastric tube

Tube inserted through the nose, down the esophagus, into the stomach.

Complications

PART SIX

Surgery

How often is surgery needed in
patients with ulcerative colitis and what operations
are typically performed?

What are the complications of surgery
for ulcerative colitis?

14. How often is surgery needed in patients with ulcerative colitis and what operations are typically performed?

Up to 30% of patients with ulcerative colitis will require surgery. Patients with pancolitis are at the highest risk of needing surgery. Surgery is usually required for the following reasons:

- Failure of medical therapy to relieve symptoms and induce remission
- Side effects of treatment become severe or life-threatening
- Megacolon (dilation of the colon that can occur in the setting of a severe attack of UC–see Question 13)
- Perforation (bursting of the colon, usually in the setting of severe colitis attack)
- Anemia (low red blood cell count related to bleeding and decrease red cell production by the bone marrow cells related to active colitis)
- Dysplasia (precancerous changes detected during colonoscopy) or colorectal cancer

Ileal pouch anal anastomosis

Operation to remove the colon and rectum. A reservoir to store the stool is created using the lower end of the small intestine (ileum) and then is joined to the anus, allowing the stool to pass normally. Also called *ileoanal pull-through operation.*

Since the 1980s, the **ileal pouch anal anastomosis (IPAA)** has become the surgical procedure of choice. In the IPAA, the entire colon and all or most of the rectum are removed (total proctocolectomy). Some surgeons remove the entire rectum (mucosectomy), while others leave one inch of the rectum in place. The surgeon then creates a reservoir using the terminal ileum (ileal pouch) to hold stool (see **Figure 10**). The ileal pouch is anastomosed (attached) to the anus or a short segment of rectum by either staples or sutures (see **Figure 11**). After an IPAA operation, the individual passes stool through the anus.

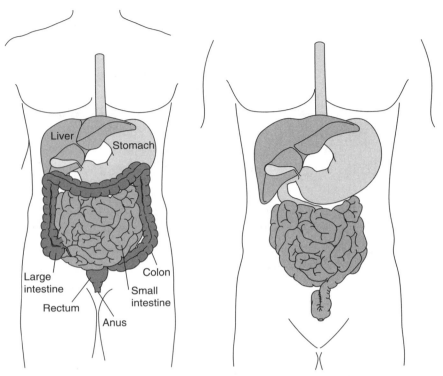

NORMAL   AFTER SURGERY

Figure 10   Normal anatomy of the intestines (L); Colon is removed and a "pouch" is created by sewing the small intestine to the anus (R).

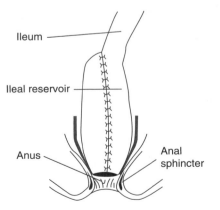

Figure 11   A pouch is created to hold the stool.

Courtesy of the National Institute of Diabetes and Digestive and Kidney Diseases.

35

In most cases a temporary ileostomy is performed. An ileostomy, an opening to the outside near your belt line at the end of the small intestine, is created by the surgeon. A bag is worn by the patient and emptied of stool several times a day. The ileostomy is usually closed 8–12 weeks after the initial surgery. There are some patients who have been undergoing one-stage IPAA, where the temporary ileostomy is not necessary. There is a higher incidence of intestinal contents leaking in the area where the intestines are attached to each other (anastomotic leak), complications from infection, and poor function in patients undergoing a one-stage IPAA. The alternative procedure to IPAA is total colectomy and permanent ileostomy. In this operation no pouch is created and the anus is permanently closed (see **Figure 12**).

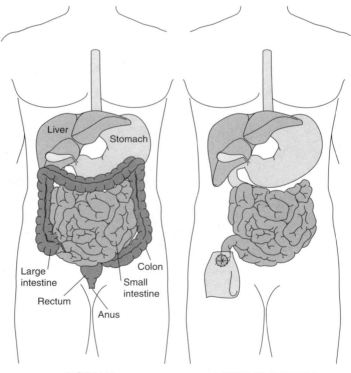

NORMAL   AFTER SURGERY

Figure 12   Normal anatomy (L); Ileostomy with bag (R).

There are different reasons for surgeons to choose each of these procedures. Patients should talk to their healthcare provider and surgeon (and consider a second opinion—see Question 19) about what is the right surgery for them. Often patients on steroid therapy, older patients, or those who need to start a weigh-loss program are not candidates for a one-stage IPAA. There are other risks and benefits to consider, and those should be discussed with a healthcare professional.

One year after successful IPAA surgery, most patients will be having 4–6 daytime bowel movements and 1 or 2 nocturnal (nighttime) bowel movements. Studies examining long term function over 10–20 years have demonstrated that patients will have an average of 4–8 bowel movements over 24 hours, with half of the patients needing to move their bowels at night. **Fecal leakage** during the day occurs in less than 4% of patients. At night the rate of seepage is 4% after 10 years and 9% 25 years after surgery. Anti-diarrheal medication is required in about a third of patients at 10 years and in 45% at 25 years.

Fecal leakage
Stool that passed through the anus without the patient's control; also called fecal incontinence.

15. What are the complications of surgery for ulcerative colitis?

Most patients are happy with their decision to have surgery for their UC; however, there can be short- and long-term complications after surgery. Short-term complications include wound infection and abscesses, both of which can be treated with antibiotics. If there are non-healing leaks around the **anastomoses** or abscesses that do not respond to antibiotics, further surgery may be necessary.

Anastomoses
Plural of anastomosis. Surgically created connection of two normally separate organs.

Surgery

Bowel obstruction

Partial or complete blockage of the small or large intestine.

Pouchitis

Inflammation of the pouch that is created after an IPAA procedure.

Long-term complications include **bowel obstruction** and inflammation of the pouch, called **pouchitis,** which is the most common complication. Bowel obstruction that does not respond to conservative measures, like placement of a nasogastric tube, may require further surgery.

PART SEVEN

Ulcerative Colitis in Older Adults

Can ulcerative colitis develop much later in life?

16. Can ulcerative colitis develop much later in life?

Although most individuals with UC are diagnosed between the ages of 15 and 30 years, about 15% of new cases of IBD are diagnosed in individuals over the age of 65 years. UC is twice as common in men if it is diagnosed after the age of 65 years. At this age, many other conditions are possible. Disorders that can present with similar symptoms of UC include ischemic colitis, colon cancer, and diverticulosis.

Diverticulosis

Common condition in which tiny pouches of tissue called diverticula poke through weak areas of the colon.

Diverticula

Plural for diverticulum, a small outpouching in the colon. These pouches are not painful and harmful unless they become inflamed. They can also lead to rectal bleeding.

Ischemic colitis occurs when blood flow is reduced to a part of the colon causing severe pain and bleeding. **Diverticulosis** is a common condition in which tiny pouches of tissue poke through weak areas in the colon. Patients with diverticulosis can develop severe rectal bleeding. If the **diverticula** become infected, the condition is called diverticulitis, which causes abdominal pain and fever.

Although treating UC in older adults is basically the same as in younger patients, there are some differences:

- Older, frail patients may have difficulty administering and retaining enema therapy
- Some studies suggest a slower response to medical therapy in older adults
- Due to an increased number of preexisting conditions in older adults, they are at an increased risk for complications and interactions with other drugs they may be taking

PART EIGHT

Coping and Surviving

Does stress cause ulcerative colitis?
Can stress affect my symptoms?

I am sick and have trouble making it to work every
day. How can I work with my employer to help them
understand my health situation?

17. Does stress cause ulcerative colitis? Can stress affect my symptoms?

Colitis was once thought to be directly related to excessive stress. Today, scientific studies have shown no increase in the risk of developing the first symptoms of IBD after a major life stress such as the loss of a job or the death of a loved one. Studies also suggest that individuals under excessive stress do not develop UC more than others.

Many patients are convinced that their colitis becomes active during stressful times in their lives. There is no question that active symptoms of colitis can create stress and when stressed, a patient can develop abdominal cramps and a tendency towards looser stools. It is important to learn the difference between abdominal pain and diarrhea caused by stress and when it is a flare-up of UC. Having diarrhea and abdominal pain does not always mean that the inflammation in your colon has worsened. It's still not clear if stress causes colonic inflammation to become worse. Regardless of the cause, efforts to reduce stress can be very helpful.

Some researchers feel that perceived stress (that is, the way that you view your own stress) is more consistently linked to an increase in symptoms of IBD. In some studies, chronic perceived stress could predict future IBD relapses, suggesting there may be a buildup of the damaging effects of stress over time.

Treatments such as **relaxation therapies, psychotherapy,** and **cognitive behavioral therapy** have been tried with IBD patients. These therapies sometimes improve well-being, coping strategies for the disease, and psychological distress, but there is as yet no objective evidence that they improve the underlying inflammation.

Relaxation therapies

Techniques such as deep breathing or imagery that allow a person to relax and relieve anxiety.

Psychotherapy

Treatment of mental or emotional problems by a therapist using a variety of communication techniques.

Cognitive-behavioral therapy

Therapeutic approach that helps individuals take control of the way they respond to illness.

Patients are encouraged to speak to their clinician about how UC is affecting their daily activities. Active disease is stressful, and psychological therapies can be helpful in coping more effectively with the distress of the disease. Some gastroenterology offices have a relationship with a psychologist or psychiatrist who has experience with patients who have to live with the stress of UC. Consider stress reduction techniques like meditation and yoga. The Crohn's and Colitis Foundation of America (CCFA) sponsors support groups throughout the country. Many individuals find comfort in speaking to others with the same condition. See the CCFA website (www.ccfa.org) for a listing of support groups in your community.

Active disease is stressful, and psychological therapies can help you cope more effectively with the distress of the disease.

It is not uncommon for UC patients to fear attacks of pain and diarrhea and be tempted to stay close to home. But, there are some things that can be done to prepare if symptoms should develop:

• Plan ahead; know the location of public restrooms. In some states, the Restroom Access Law allows access to all bathrooms in retail establishments for those having a note from their healthcare provider stating they have UC.

• If traveling on public transportation, try to sit as close to a restroom as possible.

• Carry some toilet paper, flushable wipes, and an extra set of underwear. Some people with UC may wear pads or disposable undergarments.

• Patients should consult with their clinician about taking anti-diarrheal medications at the first sign of cramping if they are not near a restroom.

When traveling further away, patients should consult with their clinician to make sure they have enough

Coping and Surviving

medication. Carrying a copy of key medical records like a colonoscopy report or CT scan report is recommended. Patients should also ask for a list of gastroenterologists who practice in the area where they are visiting.

As stress is unavoidable today, patients shouldn't hesitate to speak with their healthcare provider about methods to help with their coping skills. Finally, it is important that they understand that no matter how stressed they were before they developed colitis, the stress did not cause it.

18. I am sick and have trouble making it to work every day. How can I work with my employer to help them understand my health situation?

Patients who have a chronic illness like IBD may be covered under the Americans with Disabilities Act (ADA). They may also be eligible for time off under the Family and Medical Leave Act. The ADA has been in effect since 1992 and prohibits private employers, state and local governments, employment agencies, and labor unions from discriminating against qualified individuals with disabilities. Under the ADA, employers are required to make a "reasonable accommodation" to those with a known disability if it would not impose an "undue hardship" on the operation of the employer's business.

To be protected by the ADA, one must have a disability, which is defined as a person who has a physical or mental impairment that substantially limits one or more major life activities, a person who has a history or record of such impairment, or a person who is perceived by others as having such impairment.

An important amendment went into effect on January 1, 2009 that has a major impact on individuals with IBD. In this amendment abnormalities in gastrointestinal body functions are specifically included and are covered as a disability.

The reader is referred to the CCFA website (http://www.ccfa.org/living/disability/) for more information. Examples of "reasonable accommodations" might include:

- Allowing enough time for frequent restroom breaks
- Moving an employees' workstation closer to a restroom
- Time off or unpaid leave for doctor's appointments, flare-ups, or hospitalizations
- Providing flexible work schedules or telecommuting opportunities
- Reassignment to a different position

The Family and Medical Leave Act (FMLA) passed in 1993 provides eligible employees with a total of up to 12 work weeks of leave during a 12-month period for several reasons, including to take medical leave when the employee is unable to work because of a serious health condition. The FMLA applies to all public agencies (state, local, and federal), including schools, and to private-sector businesses that employ 50 or more employees. To be eligible, you must have been working for the same employer for at least 12 months, for at least 1,250 hours during the previous 12 months, at a location where at least 50 employees are employed by the employer within 75 miles.

Coping and Surviving

If a patient is having difficulty with their employer, they should ask their healthcare provider to write a letter describing their condition, treatment plans, and **prognosis**. Contact a local CCFA chapter or call this toll free number 1-800-932-2423 to see if they are aware of local resources including local government agencies or attorneys who are able to assist in obtaining coverage under the ADA or FMLA laws.

Prognosis

Prediction of the course of disease.

PART NINE

Future Treatments, Miscellaneous Issues, and Resources

Should I get a second opinion?

Where can I get more information about ulcerative colitis?

19. Should I get a second opinion?

Most patients with UC have mild disease that can easily be managed by a general gastroenterologist; however, some individuals have a more aggressive version of the disease. In particular, patients with extensive colitis and ongoing symptoms despite the use of steroids or immunomodulators are at increased risk for complications and might benefit from a second opinion.

Keep in mind that your healthcare provider wants you to get better and wants you to take an active role in your ongoing care. Don't be embarrassed to ask for a second opinion about treatment options, prognosis, or any aspect of their healthcare—it does not mean you don't trust your healthcare provider; it just means you want to learn more about this disease. You may be surprised to find that some healthcare insurance companies recommend or encourage patients to get second opinions. Some people choose to consult with a second healthcare provider when:

- They are considering surgery
- Their clinician prescribes a new medication
- They are not seeing an improvement in symptoms despite repeated visits to their healthcare provider
- They want to learn more about alternative treatments

There are multiple places to look when you are researching healthcare providers' credentials to find one to consult for a second opinion. Hospital websites list faculty members and their credentials. Health insurance companies have lists of resources in your community. Even your healthcare provider can suggest other clinicians for you to see. Another resource is the Crohn's and Colitis Foundation of America (www.ccfa.org) website (or call their toll-free number), which provides a list of gastroenterologists with expertise in treating IBD. Hospitals may also list information about **clinical trials** testing new medications to treat UC. If you are interested, you might be eligible to participate. Information regarding current clinical trials can be found at www.clinicaltrials.gov.

Ask your clinician to send your medical records to the physician that will be providing a second opinion. If you will be bringing the records with you, it will be helpful to have notes from office visits, results from colonoscopies, and pathology reports. Also, for reference, plan to bring along original biopsy slides, x-rays, CT, and MRI's. Prior to the appointment, the new physician may be able to provide you with a list of items they would like you to provide.

Clinical trial
Controlled research study in which human volunteers test the safety and efficacy of new drugs or treatments.

Pathology reports
Results provided by a pathologist who describes the changes seen on biopsied tissue.

Future Treatments, Miscellaneous Issues, and Resources

20. Where can I get more information about ulcerative colitis?

There are many resources available. A list of useful organizations and contact information is shown in **Table 4**. The Crohn's and Colitis Foundation of America (CCFA) has an information resource center that provides accurate, current, disease-related information. The CCFA resource center is available to the public, healthcare professionals, patients, and their families. There are local CCFA chapters throughout the country that run educational programs as well as support groups. You can find a support group near you by searching the CCFA website or calling their toll-free number. You can also search for clinical trials in your area on the CCFA website as well as at www.clinicaltrials.gov. If you provide your e-mail address to the CCFA, you can be placed on a distribution list describing advances in the field.

Table 4   Resources about Ulcerative Colitis

Name of Organization	Website	Phone No.
American College of Gastroenterology	www.acg.gi.org	301-263-9000
American Gastroenterological Association	www.gastro.org	301-654-2055
Crohn's and Colitis Foundation of America	www.ccfa.org	800-932-2423
IBD Support Foundation	www.IBDSF.com	323-938-8090
Living with UC	www.livingwithuc.com	
MyIBDCentral	www.MyIBDCentral.com	703-302-1040
National Digestive Diseases Information Clearinghouse	www2.niddk.nih.gov	800-891-5389
The Foundation for Clinical Research in IBD	www.MyIBD.org	
UC and Crohn's: A Site for Teens	www.ucandcrohns.org	
United Ostomy Association	www.uoa.org	800-826-0826

It is important for patients to talk with their clinician about food supplements or over-the-counter medications before using.

Indications

How a drug is used to treat a certain disease.

Be cautious about information found that may not be based upon medically proven claims. It is important for patients to talk with their healthcare provider about food supplements or over-the-counter medications before starting them.

Some of the drugs used to treat UC can be very expensive, but resources to pay for them are available. Pharmaceutical companies have web pages for their drugs that describe the **indications** and side effects as well as information on how to apply for support to pay for them. Other resources about assistance for paying for

specific medications include http://www.needymeds.org
(215-625-9609) or http://www.rxassist.org/search/default
.cfm (401-729-3284).

If you have insurance that requires costly co-pays, the
Patient Advocate Foundation has a program to assist
patients with ulcerative colitis (www.copays.org, or call
1-866-512-3861).

Glossary

5-ASAs: Aminosalicylates are medications used to treat the inflammation associated with ulcerative colitis; they come in oral and topical forms.

Abdominal: Related to the area between the chest and the hips containing the stomach, small intestine, large intestine, liver, gallbladder, pancreas, and spleen.

Abscess: Accumulation of pus.

Anastomosis: Surgically created connection of two normally separate organs Anastomoses (*plural*).

Anemia: Decreased red blood cells.

ANCA: Anti-neutrophil cytoplasmic antibodies detected in autoimmune disorders.

ASCA: Anti-saccharomyces cerevisiae antibody blood test detected in autoimmune disorders.

Backwash ileitis: Inflammation of the last few inches of the small intestine in patients with pancolitis.

Bifidobacteria: Naturally occurring bacteria in the human body used to treat digestive disorders.

Biologic agents: Group of therapeutic medications that include monoclonal antibodies.

Biopsy: Procedure in which a tiny piece of a body part, such as the colon or liver, is removed for examination with a microscope.

Bloating: A fullness or swelling in the abdomen.

Bowel obstruction: Partial or complete blockage of the small or large intestine.

Bowel prep: Process used to clean the colon with enemas or a special drink that causes frequent bowel movements. It is used before surgery of the colon, a colonoscopy, or a barium enema x-ray.

CBC: Abbreviation for the blood test, complete blood count, which measures red cells and white cells.

Celiac disease: Immune reaction to gluten, a protein found in wheat, rye, and barley. The disease causes damage to the lining of the small intestine and prevents absorption of nutrients. Also called *celiac sprue*, *gluten intolerance*, and *nontropical sprue*.

Chronic: Lasting for a long time.

Chromoendoscopy: Procedure by which dye is sprayed on the lining of the colon to make it easier to identify abnormalities during a colonoscopy.

Clinical trial: Controlled research study in which human volunteers test the safety and efficacy of new drugs or treatments.

Clinician: Healthcare professional engaged in the care of patients.

Cognitive-behavioral therapy: Therapeutic approach that helps individuals take control of the way they respond to illness.

Colectomy: A surgical procedure to remove all or part of the colon.

Colon: Part of the large intestine extending from the cecum to, but not including, the rectum. See *Large intestine*.

Colonoscopy: Test to look into the rectum and colon that uses a long, flexible, narrow tube with a light and tiny camera on the end. The tube is called a colonoscope.

Colorectal cancer: Cancer that starts in the colon (also called the large intestine) or the rectum (the end of the large intestine).

Corticosteroids: Class of medications given to reduce inflammation.

Crohn's disease: Form of inflammatory bowel disease that causes inflammation in the gastrointestinal (GI) tract. It usually affects the lower small intestine (also called the ileum) or the colon, but it can also affect any part of the GI tract. Also called *regional enteritis*, *granulomatous colitis*, *granulomatous colitis*, and *ileitis*. See *Inflammatory bowel disease* and *Granuloma*.

CRP: C-reactive protein is a blood test that measures a type of protein found in blood associated with inflammatory diseases and risk of heart disease.

CT scan: Abbreviation for computed tomography, a technique of imaging body organs with detailed, cross-sectional views; can be done with or without oral and intravenous contrast dye.

Diarrhea: Frequent, loose, and watery bowel movements. Causes include gastrointestinal infections, irritable bowel syndrome, inflammatory bowel disease, medicines, and malabsorption.

Distension: Stretched, expanded, or swollen out of shape.

Diverticula: Plural for diverticulum, a small outpouching in the colon. These pouches are not painful and harmful unless they become inflamed. They can also lead to rectal bleeding.

Diverticulitis: Condition that occurs when small pouches in the colon called diverticula become inflamed.

Diverticulosis: Common condition in which tiny pouches of tissue called diverticula poke through weak areas of the colon.

Double-blinded trial: Clinical trial in which neither the patient nor the clinician knows if the patient is in a treatment group or in the placebo group.

Dysplasia: Precancerous change in the lining of the gastrointestinal tract.

Enema: Insertion of a liquid into the rectum and lower colon as a treatment.

ESR: Erythrocyte sedimentation rate, a blood test that indicates inflammation in the body; it does not specify the location of the inflammation.

Extra-intestinal: Occurring outside of the intestines.

Fecal leakage: Stool that passed through the anus without the patient's control; also called fecal incontinence.

Fiber: Substance in foods that comes from plants. Fiber helps keep the stool soft so that it moves smoothly through the colon. Soluble fiber dissolves in water and is found in beans, fruit, and oat products. Insoluble fiber does not dissolve in water and is found in whole-grain products and vegetables.

Fibromyalgia: Chronic illness characterized by fatigue and widespread aching of muscles and soft tissues.

First-degree relative: Mother, father, sister, brother, son, or daughter.

Fistula: Abnormal passage between two organs, or between an organ and the outside of the body, caused when inflamed tissues come into contact and join together while healing.

Flare: Worsening of symptoms of disease.

Folate: Naturally occurring form of folic acid.

Fulminant: Rapidly developing and severe condition.

Gastroenteritis: Infection or irritation of the stomach and intestines, which may be caused by viruses or by bacteria or parasites from spoiled food or unclean water. Symptoms include diarrhea, nausea, vomiting, and abdominal cramping.

Gastroenterologist: Doctor who specializes in the diagnosis and treatment of digestive diseases.

Gastrointestinal (GI): Related to the gastrointestinal tract.

Gastrointestinal tract (GI tract): Large, muscular tube that extends from the mouth to the anus, where the movement of muscles, along with the release of hormones and enzymes, allows for the digestion of food. Also called the *alimentary canal* or *digestive tract*.

Genetic: Relating to biologic inheritance.

Gluten: Protein found in wheat, rye, and barley. In people with celiac disease, gluten damages the lining of the small intestine or causes sores on the skin. See *Celiac disease*.

Granuloma: Finding seen under the microscope in some patients with Crohn's disease.

Granulomatous colitis: Another name for Crohn's disease of the colon.

HLA-B27: Human leukocyte antigen B27, a substance controlled by Chromosome 6 that affects the immune system and is associated with ankylosing spondylitis and reactive arthritis.

Ileal pouch anal anastomosis: Operation to remove the colon and rectum. A reservoir to store the stool is created using the lower end of the small intestine (ileum) and then is joined to the anus, allowing the stool to pass normally. Also called *ileoanal pull-through operation.*

Ileitis: Inflammation of the small intestine. Many different disorders can cause inflammation of the small intestine.

Ileocolitis: Irritation of the lower part of the small intestine (ileum) and the beginning part of the colon.

Ileostomy: Operation that attaches the small intestine to an opening in the abdomen called a stoma. An ostomy pouch, attached to the stoma and worn outside the body, collects stool.

Ileum: Lower end of the small intestine.

Immune system: Complex and intertwined system of cells and genetics that controls the body's defense system against infection and other foreign organisms or substances.

Immunomodulators: Class of drugs that are capable of modifying (decrease or weaken) the effectiveness of the immune system.

Incontinence: Inability to control urination or defecation.

Indeterminate colitis: Inflammation of the colon that cannot be easily classified as either UC or CD.

Indications: How a drug is used to treat a certain disease.

Inflammation: Soreness, irritation, swelling.

Inflammatory bowel disease (IBD): Long-lasting disorders that cause inflammation in the gastrointestinal tract. The most common disorders are ulcerative colitis and Crohn's disease.

Intravenous (IV): Given into a vein.

Irritable bowel syndrome (IBS): Disorder associated with abdominal pain, bloating, and altered bowel habits. Also sometimes called *Spastic colon* or *Mucous colitis.*

Ischemic colitis: Irritation of the colon caused by decreased blood flow. It may cause bloody diarrhea.

Lactose intolerance: Being unable to digest lactose, the sugar in milk. This condition occurs when the body cannot produce lactase.

Large intestine: Part of the intestine that includes the appendix, cecum, colon, and rectum. The large intestine absorbs water from the stool and changes it from a liquid to a solid form. The large intestine is 4 feet long.

Left-sided colitis: Inflammation that extends from the rectum to the area above the sigmoid colon to the splenic flexure.

Lower bowel: Lower part of the colon that connects to the anus.

Metabolic panel: Blood tests that measure sodium, potassium, chloride, bicarbonate, blood urea nitrogen (BUN), creatinine, and glucose.

MRI scan: A magnetic resonance imaging (MRI) scan is a test that uses a magnetic field and pulses of radio wave energy to make pictures of organs and structures inside the body.

Mucosa: Lining of gastrointestinal tract organs that absorb nutrients and fluid, form a barrier, and produce mucus.

Mucosectomy: Removal of the mucosal lining of the rectum as part of an IPAA procedure.

Mucus: Clear liquid made by the intestines that coats and protects tissues in the gastrointestinal tract.

Nasogastric (NG) tube: Tube inserted through the nose, down the esophagus, into the stomach.

Nocturnal: Occurring at night.

Pancolitis: Inflammation that extends from the rectum and proximal to the splenic flexure.

Pathology reports: Results provided by a pathologist who describes the changes seen on biopsied tissue.

Perforation: Breaking open of an organ.

Polyp: An abnormal growth on the surface of the intestine.

Pouchitis: Inflammation of the pouch that is created after an IPAA procedure.

Prebiotics: Nondigestible food ingredients that are ingested by the normal bacteria occurring in the colon. They are believed to aid in digestion.

Primary sclerosing cholangitis (PSC): Irritation, scarring, and narrowing of the bile ducts inside and outside the liver. Bile builds up in the liver and may damage its cells. Many people with this condition also have ulcerative colitis.

Probiotics: Live beneficial bacteria found in food or diet supplements believed to aid in digestion.

Proctitis: Inflammation of the rectum or anus.

Proctosigmoiditis: Inflammation of the rectum and sigmoid colon.

Prognosis: Prediction of the course of disease.

Psychotherapy: Treatment of mental or emotional problems by a therapist using a variety of communication techniques.

Rectal bleeding: Bleeding that originates in the rectum and comes out through the anus.

Rectum: Lower end of the large intestine leading to the anus.

Relapse: Disease symptoms that recur after being in remission.

Relaxation therapies: Techniques such as deep breathing or imagery that allow a person to relax and relieve anxiety.

Remission: Period of time when disease does not cause symptoms.

Retention enema: Insertion of medicated fluids through the anus into the rectum and lower colon to allow the fluid to come in contact with the mucosal lining of the colon to help heal inflammation.

Rheumatologic: Having to do with diseases of the joints and connective tissues.

Sedation: Administration of medications during a test to reduce anxiety and discomfort.

Glossary

Sigmoid colon: Lower part of the colon that empties into the rectum.

Sigmoidoscopy: Looking into the sigmoid colon and rectum with a flexible or rigid tube called a sigmoidoscope.

Small bowel x-ray: X-rays of the small intestine taken as barium liquid passes through the organ. Also called *small bowel follow-through.*

Small intestine: Organ where most digestion occurs. It measures about 20 feet and includes the duodenum, jejunum, and ileum.

Splenic flexure: Sharp bend between the transverse and descending colon in the left-upper quadrant of the abdomen.

Steroid-refractory: Severe colitis that fails to respond to corticosteroids.

Stool: Solid waste that passes through the rectum as a bowel movement; includes undigested food, bacteria, mucus, and dead cells. Also called *feces.*

Superimposed: One on top of another, as in an infection on top of an existing condition.

Suppositories: Small plug of medication inserted in the rectum or vagina.

Toxic megacolon: Life-threatening complication usually from IBD that results in dilatation of the colon and possible perforation; may require emergency surgery to remove the colon.

Toxicity: The degree to which a substance can be harmful.

Tumor necrosis factor (TNF): Type of protein that promotes inflammation in the body and gastrointestinal tract.

Ulcer: Sore on the skin's surface or on the stomach or intestinal lining.

Ulcerative colitis (UC): Disease that causes ulcers and irritation in the inner lining of the colon and rectum. See *Inflammatory bowel disease.*

Ulcerative proctitis: Ulcerative colitis that occurs in the rectum.

Upper GI series: X-rays of the esophagus, stomach, and duodenum. The patient swallows barium before x-rays are taken. Barium makes the organs show up on x-rays.

Urgency: Feeling of "needing to go" (either urine or stool).

Some glossary terms are courtesy of the National Digestive Diseases Information Clearinghouse, a service of the National Institute of Diabetes and Digestive and Kidney Diseases (NIDDK), National Institutes of Health (NIH): http://digestive.niddk.nih.gov/ddiseases/pubs/dictionary/.

Index